Osteoarthritis Guide for Beginners

Exercise and Weight Management in Osteoarthritis

By

Tarquin Valen

Table of Contents

CHAPTER 1

Introduction

Osteoarthritis (OA) is a prevalent and debilitating musculoskeletal condition that significantly impacts the lives of millions of individuals worldwide. In its essence, osteoarthritis is a degenerative joint disorder characterized by the gradual breakdown of the cartilage that covers the ends of bones in the joint, leading to pain, stiffness, and reduced joint mobility. Unlike some other forms of arthritis that involve systemic inflammation, OA primarily affects the joints, particularly weight-bearing joints such as the knees, hips, and spine. It is often colloquially referred to as "wear and tear" arthritis, although the underlying mechanisms are more complex.

1.1 Definition of Osteoarthritis

Osteoarthritis is a chronic condition that develops over time as the protective cartilage that cushions the ends of bones wears down. Cartilage, a slippery and resilient tissue, normally allows smooth joint movement by preventing bones from rubbing against each other. In individuals with osteoarthritis, this cartilage gradually erodes, leading to increased friction between bones during movement. As a result, affected individuals may experience pain, swelling, and stiffness in the affected joints. Over time, the condition can progress, causing significant joint damage and affecting the overall quality of life.

The process of osteoarthritis development involves not only the breakdown of cartilage but also changes in the underlying bone, the formation of bone spurs, and inflammation of the joint lining (synovium). While it often occurs in the joints mentioned earlier, osteoarthritis can potentially affect any joint in the body. Hands, for instance, are also commonly affected, leading to difficulties in grasping and manipulating objects.

Understanding the complexities of osteoarthritis is essential for both individuals diagnosed with the condition and the broader public. It goes beyond viewing it as a natural consequence of aging; instead, recognizing osteoarthritis as a distinct medical condition helps in early identification, management, and intervention. Awareness of the risk factors, such as age, genetics, joint injuries, and obesity, can empower individuals to make informed lifestyle choices that may mitigate the onset or progression of the disease.

1.2 Importance of Understanding Osteoarthritis

Understanding osteoarthritis is crucial for several reasons. Firstly, it enables individuals to recognize the early signs and symptoms, promoting timely medical intervention. Early diagnosis allows for the implementation of effective management strategies, potentially slowing down the progression of the disease and improving overall outcomes.

Moreover, comprehension of osteoarthritis fosters informed decision-making regarding treatment options. From lifestyle modifications and physical therapy to pharmacological and surgical interventions, individuals armed with knowledge can actively participate in their healthcare, working in tandem with healthcare professionals to formulate personalized and effective treatment plans.

understanding osteoarthritis is instrumental in the prevention of the condition. By adopting a proactive approach to joint health, individuals can make lifestyle choices that reduce the risk of osteoarthritis development. This includes maintaining a healthy weight, engaging in regular physical activity, and avoiding excessive joint stress.

On a societal level, awareness of osteoarthritis is crucial for policymakers, healthcare providers, and researchers. It emphasizes the need for public health initiatives that promote joint health, allocate resources for research into new treatment modalities, and enhance accessibility to quality healthcare services for those affected by osteoarthritis.

CHAPTER 2

Understanding Osteoarthritis

Osteoarthritis (OA) is a multifaceted condition influenced by a combination of genetic, biomechanical, and environmental factors. Understanding the various aspects that contribute to the development of osteoarthritis is crucial for both individuals seeking to prevent its onset and those already diagnosed, as it informs strategies for management and intervention.

2.1 What Causes Osteoarthritis?

The causes of osteoarthritis are complex and multifactorial. While the precise etiology may vary among individuals, several common factors contribute to the development and progression of osteoarthritis.

- **Age:** One of the primary risk factors for osteoarthritis is aging. The wear and tear on joints over time can lead to the gradual deterioration of cartilage, a hallmark feature of osteoarthritis. While aging increases the susceptibility to osteoarthritis, it is not an inevitable consequence of growing older.

- **Joint Overuse or Misuse:** Repetitive stress on a particular joint or improper joint use can contribute to the development of osteoarthritis. Occupations or activities that involve frequent, intense joint movements may accelerate joint wear and tear, particularly in weight-bearing joints such as the knees and hips.

- **Joint Injury or Trauma:** Acute joint injuries, such as fractures or ligament tears, can predispose individuals to osteoarthritis. Even injuries sustained years ago can contribute to the development of osteoarthritis later in life, emphasizing the importance of proper rehabilitation and ongoing joint care.

- **Genetics:** There is a genetic component to osteoarthritis.

Individuals with a family history of the condition may be at a higher risk. Specific genetic factors can influence the integrity of joint tissues and contribute to the overall susceptibility to osteoarthritis.

- **Obesity:** Excess body weight is a significant risk factor for osteoarthritis, particularly in weight-bearing joints. The added stress on the joints in individuals with obesity can accelerate the breakdown of cartilage and increase the likelihood of osteoarthritis development.

- **Joint Congenital Abnormalities:** Some individuals may have congenital joint abnormalities that predispose them to osteoarthritis. This includes conditions where the joint structures are not formed correctly, leading to increased stress and wear on the joints.

- **Metabolic Factors:** Certain metabolic conditions, such as diabetes or hemochromatosis, may contribute to the development of osteoarthritis. Metabolic factors can affect the health of joint tissues and influence the progression of the disease.

Understanding these causative factors provides a foundation for preventive measures and targeted interventions. By addressing modifiable risk factors, individuals can take proactive steps to reduce the likelihood of osteoarthritis development and improve joint health.

2.2 Risk Factors for Osteoarthritis

While the causes of osteoarthritis contribute to its development, various risk factors increase an individual's likelihood of experiencing this condition. Recognizing these risk factors is instrumental in identifying populations at higher risk and implementing preventative measures.

- **Age:** Advanced age is a significant risk factor for osteoarthritis, with the prevalence of the condition increasing as individuals get older. The natural aging process involves changes in joint tissues, making them more susceptible to wear and tear.

- **Gender:** Osteoarthritis affects both men and women, but the risk profile varies between genders. Before the age of 45, men are more likely to develop osteoarthritis, while after 45, women have a higher prevalence. Hormonal changes, particularly during menopause, may contribute to this shift.

- **Obesity:** Excess body weight places additional stress on weight-bearing joints, such as the knees and hips, increasing the risk of osteoarthritis. Obesity is a modifiable risk factor, and weight management can play a crucial role in preventing and managing osteoarthritis.

- **Joint Injuries:** Previous joint injuries, whether from sports, accidents, or other trauma, elevate the risk of osteoarthritis.

Adequate and timely rehabilitation following joint injuries is essential to minimize this risk.

- **Genetics:** Family history and genetics play a role in osteoarthritis susceptibility. If there is a history of osteoarthritis in close family members, individuals may have a higher genetic predisposition to the condition.

- **Occupation and Joint Stress:** Certain occupations that involve repetitive joint movements, heavy lifting, or prolonged periods of standing may increase the risk of osteoarthritis. Occupational factors contributing to joint stress should be considered, and ergonomic measures can be implemented to reduce risk.

- **Joint Alignment and Structure:** The alignment and structure of joints can impact the distribution of forces across the joint surfaces. Abnormalities in joint structure or alignment may contribute to uneven wear on cartilage, leading to osteoarthritis.

- **Other Medical Conditions:** Certain medical conditions, such as rheumatoid arthritis or metabolic disorders, may increase the risk of osteoarthritis. Managing these underlying conditions is essential in preventing or minimizing the impact of osteoarthritis.

Identifying and understanding these risk factors, individuals and healthcare professionals can develop targeted prevention and management strategies. This comprehensive approach not only addresses the symptoms but also aims to modify or eliminate the factors contributing to the development and progression of osteoarthritis.

2.3 Common Symptoms of Osteoarthritis

Osteoarthritis (OA) manifests with a range of symptoms, and while the severity and progression can vary among individuals, recognizing these common signs is crucial for early detection and effective management. It's important to note that symptoms may develop gradually, and individuals may initially attribute them to normal aging or overexertion. Understanding the typical manifestations of osteoarthritis can facilitate prompt medical attention and intervention.

1. **Joint Pain:** Persistent joint pain is a hallmark symptom of osteoarthritis. This pain is often described as a deep ache or stiffness in the affected joint. Initially, it may occur during or after movement, and as the condition progresses, pain may become constant.

2. **Stiffness:** Joint stiffness, particularly after periods of inactivity such as waking up in the morning or sitting for an extended period, is a common symptom. Stiffness tends to improve with gentle movement

but may return after prolonged rest.

3. **Decreased Range of Motion:** Osteoarthritis can lead to a reduction in the range of motion in affected joints. This limitation may impact daily activities, such as bending, kneeling, or reaching.

4. **Joint Swelling:** Inflammation of the joint lining (synovium) can result in swelling. Swollen joints may feel tender and warm to the touch. While not always present, swelling can exacerbate pain and discomfort.

5. **Joint Grating or Clicking:** As cartilage wears down, the surfaces of the bones in the joint may rub against each other, resulting in a grating

sensation or audible clicking or cracking sounds during movement.

6. **Tenderness:** The affected joint may be tender to the touch. Tenderness is often localized around the joint and can be indicative of inflammation or irritation.

7. **Development of Bone Spurs:** Over time, osteoarthritis may lead to the formation of bone spurs (osteophytes) around the edges of the joint. These bony outgrowths can contribute to joint pain and affect joint function.

8. **Pain Aggravated by Weather Changes:** Some individuals with osteoarthritis report that changes in weather conditions,

especially cold and damp weather, can exacerbate joint pain.

9. **Difficulty in Activities of Daily Living:** As osteoarthritis progresses, individuals may find it challenging to perform everyday tasks, such as walking, climbing stairs, or gripping objects. This can significantly impact quality of life.

10. **Fatigue:** Chronic pain and dealing with the limitations imposed by osteoarthritis can contribute to fatigue. The emotional toll of managing a chronic condition may also play a role in feelings of tiredness.

It's important to recognize that the symptoms of osteoarthritis can vary depending on the affected joint(s) and the stage of the condition. While there is no cure for osteoarthritis, early diagnosis and appropriate management strategies, including lifestyle modifications, physical therapy, and medication, can help alleviate symptoms, slow down the progression of the disease, and improve overall joint function and quality of life. If individuals experience persistent joint symptoms, seeking medical attention for an accurate diagnosis and tailored treatment plan is crucial.

CHAPTER 3

Diagnosis

Timely and accurate diagnosis of osteoarthritis (OA) is essential for effective management and intervention. While healthcare professionals play a pivotal role in the diagnostic process, individuals should also be aware of the symptoms that may indicate the presence of osteoarthritis. Recognizing these symptoms can prompt individuals to seek medical attention, leading to a thorough evaluation and appropriate diagnosis.

3.1 Recognizing Symptoms

Recognizing the symptoms of osteoarthritis involves paying attention to changes in joint health and functionality. The following are key symptoms that may indicate the presence of osteoarthritis:

1. **Joint Pain:** Persistent or recurring pain in one or more joints, particularly during or after movement, is a primary symptom of osteoarthritis. The pain may be described as a deep ache or stiffness.

2. **Stiffness:** Joint stiffness, especially after periods of inactivity, is a common early sign of osteoarthritis. Stiffness typically improves with gentle movement but may return after prolonged rest.

3. **Decreased Range of Motion:**
   Difficulty or limitation in the
   ability to move a joint through
   its full range of motion can be
   indicative of osteoarthritis. This
   may manifest as difficulty
   bending, kneeling, or reaching.

4. **Joint Swelling:** Inflammation
   of the joint lining can lead to
   swelling. Swollen joints may
   appear puffy and feel tender to
   the touch. Swelling is not
   always present but can
   contribute to pain and
   discomfort.

5. **Joint Grating or Clicking:**
   Sensations of joint grating,
   clicking, or cracking sounds
   during movement may indicate
   the erosion of cartilage and
   bone rubbing against each
   other.

6. **Tenderness:** Tenderness around the joint, especially when applying pressure, can be a sign of inflammation or irritation in the joint.

7. **Difficulty in Activities of Daily Living:** Challenges in performing everyday tasks, such as walking, climbing stairs, or gripping objects, may suggest the impact of osteoarthritis on joint function.

8. **Fatigue:** Chronic pain and the physical limitations imposed by osteoarthritis can contribute to feelings of fatigue. Emotional stress related to managing a chronic condition may also play a role.

9. **Pain Aggravated by Weather Changes:** Some individuals

with osteoarthritis report that changes in weather conditions, particularly cold and damp weather, can worsen joint pain.

10. **Development of Bone Spurs:** In advanced stages, the formation of bone spurs around the edges of the joint may contribute to pain and affect joint function.

Individuals who experience persistent or worsening joint symptoms should consult with a healthcare professional. A thorough medical history, physical examination, and diagnostic tests, such as X-rays or MRI scans, may be conducted to confirm the presence of osteoarthritis, assess its severity, and rule out other possible causes of joint symptoms.

It's important to note that early intervention is key to managing osteoarthritis effectively. Seeking medical advice allows for the development of a personalized treatment plan that may include lifestyle modifications, physical therapy, medications, and other interventions aimed at improving joint function and relieving symptoms. Regular follow-ups with healthcare providers ensure ongoing monitoring and adjustments to the treatment plan as needed.

3.2 Medical Tests and Diagnosis

Diagnosing osteoarthritis (OA) involves a comprehensive approach, combining clinical evaluation, medical history assessment, and various diagnostic tests. Healthcare professionals use these tools to confirm the presence of osteoarthritis, determine its severity, and develop an individualized treatment plan. Here are the key components of the medical tests and diagnostic process for osteoarthritis:

1. **Medical History:**

   - **Symptom Assessment:** The healthcare provider will inquire about the nature, duration, and intensity of joint symptoms, including pain, stiffness, and swelling.

   - **Previous Injuries or Surgeries:** Any history of joint injuries, surgeries, or other medical conditions that may contribute to joint symptoms will be explored.

2. **Physical Examination:**

- **Joint Assessment:** The healthcare professional will physically examine the affected joint(s), assessing for tenderness, swelling, range of motion, and signs of deformity.

- **Gait Analysis:** Observing how an individual walks (gait analysis) can provide insights into joint function and detect any abnormal patterns

associated with
osteoarthritis.

3. **Imaging Studies:**

- **X-rays:** X-rays are
commonly used to
visualize the bones and
joints. They can reveal
joint space narrowing,
bone spurs, and other
structural changes
characteristic of
osteoarthritis.

- **MRI (Magnetic
Resonance Imaging):** In
some cases, MRI scans
may be ordered to
provide a more detailed
view of the soft tissues,
such as cartilage and
ligaments, in and around
the joint.

4. **Joint Aspiration (Arthrocentesis):**

- In certain situations, a healthcare provider may perform joint aspiration to remove a small sample of synovial fluid from the affected joint. Analyzing this fluid can help rule out other joint-related conditions, such as inflammatory arthritis.

5. **Blood Tests:**

- Blood tests are not typically used to diagnose osteoarthritis, as it is not primarily an inflammatory condition. However, they may be ordered to rule out other forms of arthritis, such as rheumatoid arthritis, which involve systemic inflammation.

6. **Clinical Criteria:**

- Healthcare professionals often use established clinical criteria, such as those from the American College of Rheumatology, to aid in the diagnosis of osteoarthritis. These criteria consider a combination of clinical symptoms, physical examination findings, and imaging results.

It's important to note that there is no single definitive test for osteoarthritis, and the diagnosis is typically based on a combination of clinical judgment and supporting evidence from imaging and other tests. Additionally, the diagnostic process may vary depending on the affected joint and the individual's overall health.

Once a diagnosis is confirmed, the healthcare provider works collaboratively with the individual to develop a comprehensive treatment plan. This plan may include lifestyle modifications, physical therapy, pain management strategies, and, in some cases, surgical interventions. Regular follow-ups and ongoing communication with healthcare providers are essential for monitoring the progression of osteoarthritis and adjusting the treatment plan as needed to optimize joint health and overall well-being.

CHAPTER 4

Types of Osteoarthritis

Osteoarthritis (OA) is a diverse condition that can affect various joints in the body, and the manifestation of the disease can vary depending on the specific joint involved. Understanding the types of osteoarthritis, both in terms of general characteristics and specific joint involvement, is crucial for accurate diagnosis and targeted management.

4.1 General Overview

Osteoarthritis is a degenerative joint disorder characterized by the gradual breakdown of cartilage in the joints. This breakdown leads to changes in the underlying bone, the formation of bone spurs, and, in some cases, inflammation of the joint lining. While it can affect any joint in the body, certain joints are more commonly impacted, including:

- **Knees:** Osteoarthritis of the knee is one of the most prevalent forms of the condition. It often results in pain, stiffness, and reduced range of motion, making activities like walking or climbing stairs challenging.

- **Hips:** Osteoarthritis in the hip joints can cause pain and stiffness, particularly during movement. As the condition progresses, individuals may experience difficulty with activities like walking or

getting up from a seated
position.

- **Spine:** Osteoarthritis can affect
the spine, including the neck
(cervical spine) and the lower
back (lumbar spine). Symptoms
may include pain, stiffness,
and, in some cases, radiating
pain or numbness into the
extremities.

- **Hands and Fingers:**
Osteoarthritis in the hands and
fingers can lead to joint pain,
stiffness, and difficulties with
fine motor tasks. The formation
of small, bony outgrowths,
known as Heberden's nodes and
Bouchard's nodes, is
characteristic of hand
osteoarthritis.

- **Feet and Toes:** While less common, osteoarthritis can also affect the joints of the feet and toes. This can result in pain, swelling, and difficulty with walking.

- **Shoulders:** Osteoarthritis of the shoulder joints may cause pain and reduced range of motion, particularly when lifting or rotating the arm.

- **Other Joints:** Osteoarthritis can potentially affect any joint, including those in the elbows, wrists, and ankles, although these instances are less frequent.

4.2 Specific Joint Involvement

Each type of osteoarthritis may present unique challenges and require tailored management strategies:

- **Knee Osteoarthritis:** Common symptoms include knee pain, stiffness, and difficulty bending or straightening the knee. Lifestyle modifications, physical therapy, and, in severe cases, surgical options like knee replacement may be considered.

- **Hip Osteoarthritis:** Symptoms often include hip pain, stiffness, and reduced hip joint mobility. Treatment may involve pain management, exercise, and, in advanced cases, hip replacement surgery.

- **Hand Osteoarthritis:** Individuals with hand osteoarthritis may experience pain, swelling, and difficulties with gripping or manipulating objects. Treatment options include joint protection techniques, medications, and hand exercises.

- **Spinal Osteoarthritis (Spondylosis):** Symptoms can include back pain, stiffness, and, in some cases, nerve-related symptoms if the spinal nerves are affected. Management may involve physical therapy, pain medication, and lifestyle adjustments.

- **Foot and Toe Osteoarthritis:** Pain, swelling, and difficulty with walking or wearing certain shoes are common symptoms. Footwear modifications, orthotics, and physical therapy may be recommended.

Understanding the specific joint involvement allows healthcare professionals to tailor interventions to address the unique challenges of each case. It also empowers individuals with osteoarthritis to actively participate in their care by adopting strategies that specifically target the affected joints. Early diagnosis and proactive management are key in mitigating the impact of osteoarthritis on joint function and overall quality of life.

CHAPTER 5

Treatment Options

Managing osteoarthritis (OA) involves a multifaceted approach that combines lifestyle modifications, medications, and other interventions to alleviate symptoms, improve joint function, and enhance overall quality of life. The choice of treatment options often depends on the severity of the condition, the specific joints affected, and individual health considerations.

5.1 Lifestyle Changes

Lifestyle modifications play a crucial role in the management of osteoarthritis, focusing on improving joint health and reducing the impact of symptoms.

1. **Weight Management:**

   - Maintaining a healthy weight is paramount, especially for weight-bearing joints like the knees and hips. Weight loss can significantly reduce stress on joints, alleviate pain, and slow down the progression of osteoarthritis.

2. **Exercise:**

   - Regular, low-impact exercise is beneficial for joint health. Activities such as walking, swimming, and cycling help maintain joint flexibility, strengthen supporting muscles, and manage weight. Consultation with a healthcare provider or a physical therapist can guide the development of an appropriate exercise plan.

3. **Joint Protection Techniques:**

- Implementing joint protection strategies during daily activities can help reduce strain on joints. This may include using assistive devices, ergonomic tools, and avoiding excessive repetitive movements.

4. **Balanced Diet:**

- A balanced and nutritious diet supports

overall health, including joint health. Omega-3 fatty acids, found in fish and certain nuts, have anti-inflammatory properties that may benefit individuals with osteoarthritis.

5. **Heat and Cold Therapy:**

- Applying heat or cold to affected joints can provide symptomatic relief. Heat helps relax muscles and ease stiffness, while cold reduces inflammation and numbs pain. This can be achieved through warm compresses, ice packs, or topical creams.

6. **Physical Therapy:**

- Physical therapists can design customized exercise programs to improve joint flexibility, strength, and range of motion. They also teach individuals proper body mechanics and techniques for managing daily activities with minimal joint stress.

5.2 Medications

Various medications are used to manage pain, reduce inflammation, and improve joint function in individuals with osteoarthritis.

1. **Analgesics (Pain Relievers):**

   - Over-the-counter pain relievers such as

acetaminophen can help
alleviate mild to
moderate pain associated
with osteoarthritis.
Prescription-strength
pain relievers, such as
tramadol, may be
considered for more
severe pain.

2. **Nonsteroidal Anti-Inflammatory Drugs (NSAIDs):**

   - NSAIDs, available over-the-counter or by prescription, can help reduce pain and inflammation. Common NSAIDs include ibuprofen and naproxen. However, long-term use may have potential side effects, so their use should be monitored by a healthcare provider.

3. **Topical Analgesics:**

   - Creams, gels, or patches containing topical analgesics, such as NSAIDs or capsaicin, can be applied directly to the skin over the affected joint to provide localized pain relief.

4. **Corticosteroid Injections:**

   - Intra-articular corticosteroid injections may be recommended for individuals with significant joint inflammation. These injections deliver anti-inflammatory medication directly into the joint, providing targeted relief.

5. **Hyaluronic Acid Injections:**

   - In some cases, injections of hyaluronic acid, a substance that lubricates and cushions the joint, may be considered. This treatment aims to improve joint mobility and reduce pain.

6. **Disease-Modifying Osteoarthritis Drugs (DMOADs):**

   - Research is ongoing in the development of disease-modifying drugs that target specific pathways involved in the progression of osteoarthritis. These drugs aim to slow down joint degeneration and modify the course of the disease.

Individuals with osteoarthritis should work closely with their healthcare team to determine the most appropriate treatment plan based on their symptoms, overall health, and the specific joints affected. It's important to note that treatment strategies may evolve over time, and regular follow-ups with healthcare providers help ensure that the management plan remains effective and is adjusted as needed.

5.3 Physical Therapy

Physical therapy is a key component of the comprehensive treatment approach for osteoarthritis. It focuses

*on improving joint function, relieving
pain, and enhancing overall mobility
through targeted exercises and
therapeutic interventions.*

1. **Exercise Programs:**

    - Physical therapists
      design tailored exercise
      programs that address
      specific joint limitations
      and muscle weaknesses.
      These programs typically
      include a combination of
      flexibility, strength
      training, and aerobic
      exercises to improve
      joint stability and
      function.

2. **Joint Range of Motion
    Exercises:**

    - Range of motion
      exercises aim to enhance

the flexibility of affected
joints. These exercises
may involve gentle
stretches and controlled
movements to promote
optimal joint mobility.

3. **Strength Training:**

- Strengthening exercises
  target the muscles
  surrounding the affected
  joint. Building muscle
  strength helps provide
  better support to the
  joints, reducing stress
  and improving overall
  joint function.

4. **Low-Impact Aerobic Exercises:**

- Activities such as
  swimming, cycling, and
  walking are

recommended as they
promote cardiovascular
health without placing
excessive stress on the
joints. Aerobic exercises
also contribute to weight
management.

5. **Manual Therapy:**

   - Manual therapy
     techniques, such as joint
     mobilization and
     manipulation, are
     administered by physical
     therapists to alleviate
     joint stiffness, improve
     range of motion, and
     reduce pain.

6. **Assistive Devices and
   Techniques:**

   - Physical therapists may
     recommend the use of

assistive devices, such as braces or splints, to support and stabilize affected joints. They also educate individuals on proper body mechanics to minimize joint stress during daily activities.

7. **Pain Management Strategies:**

- Physical therapists employ various pain management techniques, including heat or cold therapy, ultrasound, and electrical stimulation, to alleviate pain and improve comfort during therapy sessions.

8. **Education and Lifestyle Guidance:**

- Education is a crucial aspect of physical therapy. Individuals receive guidance on joint protection, proper posture, and lifestyle modifications that can positively impact their overall joint health.

Physical therapy is particularly beneficial in the early stages of osteoarthritis, but it can also provide valuable support at any stage of the condition. Regular sessions with a physical therapist, combined with adherence to recommended home exercises, contribute to sustained joint health and functional improvement.

CHAPTER 6

Pain Management

6.1 Alternative Therapies

In addition to conventional medical treatments, various alternative therapies can complement the management of osteoarthritis by providing additional avenues for pain relief, improved joint function, and enhanced overall well-being. It's essential to note that individual responses to alternative therapies can vary, and it's advisable to consult with healthcare professionals before incorporating them into a treatment plan.

1. **Physical Modalities:**

- **Physical Therapy:**
  Structured physical
  therapy programs, as
  discussed earlier, focus
  on targeted exercises to
  improve joint function,
  alleviate pain, and
  enhance mobility.
  Physical therapists may
  incorporate techniques
  such as ultrasound or
  electrical stimulation to
  further support pain
  relief.

2. **Mind-Body Practices:**

- **Yoga:** Yoga combines
  physical postures,
  breathing exercises, and
  meditation. It can
  improve flexibility,
  strength, and balance,
  while also promoting

relaxation and stress reduction.

- **Tai Chi:** Tai Chi is a gentle Chinese martial art that emphasizes slow, flowing movements. It has been shown to improve balance, reduce pain, and enhance overall well-being in individuals with osteoarthritis.

3. **Manual Therapies:**

- **Massage Therapy:** Massage can help reduce muscle tension, improve circulation, and provide temporary relief from joint pain. It's essential to choose a massage therapist experienced in working with individuals with osteoarthritis.

- **Chiropractic Care:** Chiropractors may use manual adjustments to improve joint alignment and alleviate pain. However, caution is advised, and individuals should ensure that chiropractic care is coordinated with their overall healthcare plan.

4. **Acupuncture:**

- Acupuncture involves the insertion of thin needles into specific points on the body. Some individuals with osteoarthritis report pain relief and improved joint function with acupuncture. It's important to seek acupuncture from qualified and licensed practitioners.

5. **Nutritional Supplements:**

- **Glucosamine and Chondroitin:** These are commonly used dietary supplements that are believed to support joint health. While research results are mixed, some individuals report benefits in terms of reduced pain and improved function. Consultation with a healthcare provider is recommended before starting these supplements.

- **Omega-3 Fatty Acids:** Found in fish oil supplements, omega-3 fatty acids have anti-inflammatory properties and may offer some relief from joint pain. However, their efficacy can vary among individuals.

6. **Heat and Cold Therapy:**

- **Heat Packs and Warm Baths:** Applying heat to affected joints can help relax muscles and alleviate stiffness. Warm baths, hot packs, or heated blankets may provide relief.

- **Cold Packs:** Cold therapy can reduce inflammation and numb pain. Cold packs or ice packs applied to the affected joint may be beneficial.

7. **Herbal Remedies:**

- **Turmeric and Boswellia:** These herbs have anti-inflammatory properties and are believed by some to reduce joint pain. However, evidence is limited, and individuals should consult with healthcare providers before using herbal supplements.

8. **Weight Management Programs:**

- For individuals with osteoarthritis in weight-bearing joints, programs focused on weight management and healthy lifestyle choices can contribute to reduced joint stress and improved overall joint health.

It's important to approach alternative therapies with a well-informed and cautious mindset. While some individuals find relief through these approaches, scientific evidence supporting their efficacy can vary, and results may be subjective. Before incorporating alternative therapies into a treatment plan, individuals should discuss their intentions with healthcare providers to ensure compatibility with overall care and to address any potential interactions or contraindications. Additionally, ongoing communication with healthcare professionals is crucial to monitor the effectiveness of alternative therapies in the context of managing osteoarthritis.

CHAPTER 7

Living with Osteoarthritis

7.1 Coping Strategies for Living with Osteoarthritis

Living with osteoarthritis can present various challenges, both physical and emotional. Adopting effective coping strategies is essential for managing symptoms, maintaining quality of life, and promoting overall well-being. Here are some coping strategies that individuals with osteoarthritis may find beneficial:

1. **Education and Self-Management:**

- **Knowledge is Empowerment:** Learn as much as possible about osteoarthritis, including its causes, symptoms, and available treatments. Understanding the condition empowers individuals to actively participate in their care and make informed decisions.

2. **Pain Management Techniques:**

- **Heat and Cold Therapy:** Use heat packs, warm baths, or cold packs to manage joint pain and stiffness.

- **Topical Analgesics:**
  Apply topical creams or
  patches containing
  analgesic ingredients
  directly to the affected
  joints for localized pain
  relief.

- **Mind-Body Practices:**
  Engage in relaxation
  techniques, such as deep
  breathing or meditation,
  to manage pain and
  reduce stress.

3. **Adopting a Healthy Lifestyle:**

   - **Regular Exercise:**
     Follow a tailored
     exercise plan designed
     by a healthcare
     professional or physical
     therapist. Low-impact
     activities, such as

walking or swimming, can help maintain joint function.

- **Balanced Diet:** Consume a nutritious diet rich in fruits, vegetables, lean proteins, and whole grains. Omega-3 fatty acids, found in fish and certain nuts, may have anti-inflammatory effects.

- **Weight Management:** Maintain a healthy weight to reduce stress on weight-bearing joints, such as the knees and hips.

4. **Joint Protection Techniques:**

- **Proper Body Mechanics:** Learn and

practice techniques for minimizing stress on the joints during daily activities. This includes using assistive devices and avoiding repetitive movements that may exacerbate symptoms.

5. **Assistive Devices and Home Modifications:**

   - **Use of Braces or Splints:** Assistive devices can provide support to affected joints and improve stability.

   - **Home Modifications:** Consider making modifications at home, such as installing handrails or ramps, to enhance accessibility and safety.

6. **Social Support:**

   - **Join Support Groups:** Connecting with others who are also living with osteoarthritis can provide emotional support, shared experiences, and practical tips for managing the condition.

   - **Family and Friends:** Communicate openly with loved ones about your needs and challenges. Seek their understanding and enlist their support in your journey.

7. **Mind-Body Practices:**

- **Mindfulness and Relaxation:** Practices such as mindfulness meditation and progressive muscle relaxation can help manage stress and improve overall well-being.

- **Counseling or Therapy:** Professional counseling can provide valuable emotional support and coping strategies for dealing with the emotional aspects of living with a chronic condition.

8. **Regular Healthcare Monitoring:**

- **Follow-Up with Healthcare Providers:** Attend regular check-ups and follow-ups with healthcare professionals to monitor the progression of osteoarthritis and adjust treatment plans as needed.

9. **Adaptive Strategies:**

- **Modify Activities:** Adapt daily activities to accommodate the limitations imposed by osteoarthritis. Break tasks into smaller, manageable steps, and pace yourself.

- **Plan and Prioritize:** Plan activities based on

energy levels and prioritize tasks to avoid overexertion.

10. **Maintaining a Positive Outlook:**

- **Focus on What You Can Do:** Emphasize and celebrate the activities you can still enjoy rather than dwelling on limitations.

- **Set Realistic Goals:** Establish achievable goals that align with your abilities, fostering a sense of accomplishment.

Coping with osteoarthritis is a dynamic process that may require ongoing adjustment and the incorporation of new strategies over time. Tailoring coping strategies to individual needs and seeking professional guidance, when necessary, can contribute to a more effective and positive approach to managing osteoarthritis.

7.2 Exercise and Weight Management in Osteoarthritis

Effective management of osteoarthritis often involves a combination of exercise and weight management strategies. These approaches aim to improve joint function, alleviate symptoms, and enhance overall well-being. Here's an overview of how exercise and weight management play crucial roles in managing osteoarthritis:

Exercise:

1. **Benefits of Exercise:**

   - **Joint Flexibility:**
     Regular exercise helps
     maintain and improve
     joint flexibility, reducing
     stiffness and promoting
     better range of motion.

   - **Muscle Strengthening:**
     Strengthening the
     muscles around affected
     joints provides added
     support, reducing stress
     on the joints and
     improving overall joint
     stability.

   - **Weight Management:**
     Exercise contributes to
     weight management,
     which is particularly
     important for individuals

with osteoarthritis in weight-bearing joints.

2. **Types of Exercise for Osteoarthritis:**

- **Low-Impact Aerobic Exercises:** Activities such as walking, swimming, and cycling are gentle on the joints while providing cardiovascular benefits.

- **Strength Training:** Targeted strength training exercises focus on building muscle around the affected joints. This can be done with resistance bands, weights, or bodyweight exercises.

- **Range of Motion Exercises:** Gentle stretches and range of motion exercises help maintain flexibility and prevent joint stiffness.

- **Water Exercise:** Aquatic exercises in a pool reduce the impact on joints while providing resistance for muscle strengthening.

3. **Exercise Guidelines:**

- **Consultation with Healthcare Providers:** Before starting an exercise program, individuals should consult with their healthcare providers to ensure that the chosen activities are safe and appropriate for their specific condition.

- **Gradual Progression:** Start slowly and gradually increase the intensity and duration of exercise. This approach minimizes the risk of injury and allows the body to adapt.

- **Consistency:** Consistency is key to experiencing the long-term benefits of exercise. Regular, moderate-intensity exercise is generally more beneficial than sporadic, high-intensity activities.

4. **Adaptive Exercise Strategies:**

- **Modify Activities:**
  Adapt exercises to
  accommodate joint
  limitations. For example,
  choose low-impact
  alternatives and avoid
  activities that exacerbate
  pain.

- **Balance Exercises:**
  Incorporate exercises that
  improve balance, as
  individuals with
  osteoarthritis may be at
  an increased risk of falls.

Weight Management:

1. **Importance of Weight
   Management:**

   - **Reduced Joint Stress:**
     Maintaining a healthy
     weight is crucial for
     individuals with

osteoarthritis, especially in weight-bearing joints like the knees and hips. Excess weight places additional stress on joints, contributing to pain and the progression of the condition.

- **Improved Joint Function:** Weight loss can lead to improved joint function and increased mobility, enhancing overall quality of life.

2. **Weight Management Strategies:**

- **Balanced Diet:** Adopt a balanced and nutritious diet that includes a variety of fruits, vegetables, lean proteins, and whole grains. Limit the intake of processed foods, sugary beverages, and excessive amounts of saturated fats.

- **Portion Control:** Be mindful of portion sizes to avoid overeating. Smaller, more frequent meals may be beneficial.

- **Hydration:** Drink an adequate amount of water, as staying hydrated is important for overall health and can help control appetite.

- **Regular Physical Activity:** Engage in regular physical activity to burn calories and support weight management.

3. **Professional Guidance:**

- **Consultation with Healthcare Providers or Dietitians:** Seeking guidance from healthcare providers or registered dietitians can help individuals develop personalized nutrition plans that align with their health goals and dietary needs.

- **Behavioral Support:** For some individuals, behavioral support from healthcare professionals or support groups can be beneficial in addressing emotional and behavioral

aspects of weight
management.

4. **Long-Term Lifestyle
    Changes:**

    - **Sustainable
      Approaches:** Focus on
      sustainable lifestyle
      changes rather than
      short-term diets.
      Adopting habits that are
      realistic and maintainable
      contributes to long-term
      success.

5. **Monitor Progress:**

    - **Regular Monitoring:**
      Regularly monitor
      weight and assess
      progress. Celebrate
      achievements and make
      adjustments to the plan
      as needed.

Incorporating regular exercise and weight management strategies into a comprehensive osteoarthritis management plan, individuals can actively contribute to improved joint health, reduced pain, and enhanced overall well-being. It's crucial to approach these lifestyle changes with patience, consistency, and a focus on long-term health benefits.

7.3 Encouragement for Those Living with Osteoarthritis

Living with osteoarthritis can be challenging, both physically and emotionally. However, with the right mindset, support, and proactive management, individuals with osteoarthritis can lead fulfilling lives. Here's a message of encouragement for those navigating the journey of osteoarthritis:

1. **You Are Not Alone:**

   - Osteoarthritis affects millions of people worldwide. Remember that you are not alone in facing the challenges posed by this condition. Many individuals share similar experiences and can offer support and understanding.

2. **Celebrating Small Victories:**

   - Every achievement, no matter how small, deserves recognition. Celebrate the victories, whether it's completing an exercise routine, managing pain more effectively, or adapting successfully to daily challenges. Each step forward is a testament to your strength and resilience.

3. **Your Journey, Your Pace:**

- Osteoarthritis is a unique journey for each person. Embrace the pace that works for you. It's not about racing to the finish line but about making consistent, sustainable progress that enhances your overall well-being.

4. **Focus on What You Can Do:**

- While osteoarthritis may introduce limitations, it's essential to focus on what you can do rather

than what you can't.
Adapting activities,
setting realistic goals,
and exploring new
interests can bring a
sense of accomplishment
and joy.

5. **Building a Support Network:**

*   Surround yourself with a
    supportive network of
    friends, family,
    healthcare professionals,
    and fellow individuals
    facing osteoarthritis.
    Share your experiences,
    seek advice, and draw
    strength from those who
    understand and
    empathize.

6. **Mind-Body Connection:**

- Acknowledge the mind-body connection. Practices such as mindfulness, meditation, and deep breathing can help manage stress and improve overall well-being. Taking care of your mental health is an integral part of managing osteoarthritis.

7. **Adapting to Change:**

- Osteoarthritis may bring changes to your daily life, but it also presents opportunities for adaptation and growth. Embrace the journey of finding new ways to navigate challenges and discover what brings joy and fulfillment.

8. **Communication with Healthcare Providers:**

- Open communication
  with healthcare providers
  is crucial. Share your
  concerns, ask questions,
  and actively participate
  in your healthcare
  decisions. A
  collaborative approach
  ensures that your
  treatment plan is tailored
  to your unique needs.

9. **Learning and Empowerment:**

- Knowledge is a powerful
  tool. Educate yourself
  about osteoarthritis,
  treatment options, and
  self-management
  strategies. Being
  informed empowers you

to actively engage in your care and advocate for the best possible outcomes.

10. **Patience and Self-Compassion:**

- Be patient with yourself. Osteoarthritis management is a journey, and progress may take time. Cultivate self-compassion, recognizing that you are doing your best in the face of challenges.

11. **Seeking Joy in Everyday Moments:**

- Amidst the challenges, find joy in simple, everyday moments. Whether it's enjoying a

favorite activity,
spending time with loved
ones, or appreciating the
beauty around you,
cultivating a positive
mindset can make a
significant difference.

Living with osteoarthritis is about
embracing the fullness of life despite
the challenges it may present. Each
day is an opportunity for growth,
resilience, and finding moments of
joy. You have the strength to navigate
this journey, and your unique
experiences contribute to a narrative
of courage and perseverance.

www.ingramcontent.com/pod-product-compliance
Lightning Source LLC
Chambersburg PA
CBHW050831260726
48660CB00006B/2184